D0723651

It's Not About the Boobs!

FINDING HUMOR IN HEALING

Note for Librarians: A cataloguing record for this book is available from Library and Archives Canada at www.collectionscanada.ca/amicus/index-e.html

ISBN 1-4120-6983-1

Printed in Victoria, BC, Canada. Printed on paper with minimum 30% recycled fibre. Trafford's print shop runs on "green energy" from solar, wind and other environmentally-friendly power sources.

TRAFFORD
PUBLISHING™

Offices in Canada, USA, Ireland and UK
This book was published on-demand in cooperation with Trafford Publishing. On-demand publishing is a unique process and service of making a book available for retail sale to the public taking advantage of on-demand manufacturing and Internet marketing. On-demand publishing includes promotions, retail sales, manufacturing, order fulfilment, accounting and collecting royalties on behalf of the author.

Book sales for North America and international:
Trafford Publishing, 6E–2333 Government St.,
Victoria, BC V8T 4P4 CANADA
phone 250 383 6864 (toll-free 1 888 232 4444)
fax 250 383 6804; email to orders@trafford.com
Book sales in Europe:
Trafford Publishing (UK) Limited, 9 Park End Street, 2nd Floor
Oxford, UK 0x1 1HH UNITED KINGDOM
phone 44 (0)1865 722 113 (local rate 0845 230 9601)
facsimile 44 (0)1865 722 868; info.uk@trafford.com
Order online at:
trafford.com/05-1894

10 9 8 7 6 5 4 3 2

DEDICATION

To my Mom who cared for my kids while I was sick. I don't even want to imagine how awful it was to see your child so ill, and to feel so helpless.

To my family, I have never felt more love and support. I am truly blessed.

To my brother Matt, you kept me sane when no one else could. You're the best brother.

To my kids, you fulfill my life and give me purpose.

To my support group ladies, if you only knew how grateful I am to know you. You are my super heroes. Thank you Maria.

To my doctors, I am the luckiest patient in the world. You are truly blessed with the gift of caring.

To my husband P.J., you are my rock. I love you so much. You give me hope when I waiver in my faith. You think I'm beautiful no matter what.

Most important, to God. Just the thought of what you endured for me, gives me the strength to fight and be a better person.

INTRODUCTION

Well where do I begin. A lot of people have told me to write my story down. Unfortunately, it's really no different from the many women who get the terrible news that they have breast cancer. Especially the horror that they go through. But perhaps how I choose to deal with it is. Some of you might not understand why I choose to deal with it in this way but this is who I am. My motto is, that out of something bad you can find good. And humor is my savior. Of course so is God.

So humor softens the blow and faith does the healing. I don't want to be misunderstood. Cancer is no laughing matter and I don't take it lightly. Am I glad I have cancer? Well of course not. Am I a better person because of it? Yes. Do I think God gave me cancer? No! Do I think he wants me to do something good with this? Yes. And maybe just telling my story is a start.

I was thirty-four when I was diagnosed with advanced breast cancer. I have a husband and two children. And unfortunately, it took me to be diagnosed with cancer to see that I took all of them for granted. Cancer is quite humbling. It reminds us of how human we really are. When I was diagnosed, my world stopped. I was in a daze for about three weeks. I t was absolute despair. That was roughly the time it took for all my tests to be done and results to come in. It was torture. My fear was that I wouldn't see my children grow up. I was

7

angry. More angry than scared. It was the purest anger that I had ever felt. But something told me to snap out of it. Pull yourself together that I wasn't a statistic. Nobody would make me a number. Things began to change for me then. I found beauty in things I never paid attention too before. I didn't take things for granted. Most importantly I started to smile and laugh again. Laughing is wonderful. I even took that for granted. I realized that the more I laughed and joked around the better I felt mentally. I became more approachable. People felt like they could ask me questions about my diagnosis, cancer itself. I thought perhaps there's something more to this. I was tired of crying so I decided to start laughing. I found humor in every aspect of my treatment. And it helps me to stay positive to this day. That's when I decided I should start writing this stuff down. Maybe I could cheer some people up. My only hope is that it will make you laugh, smile and maybe take your mind off the bad things for a while.

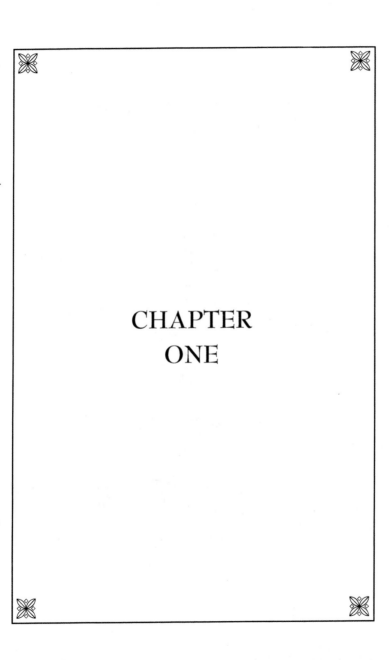

CHAPTER
ONE

DIAGNOSING AND STAGING

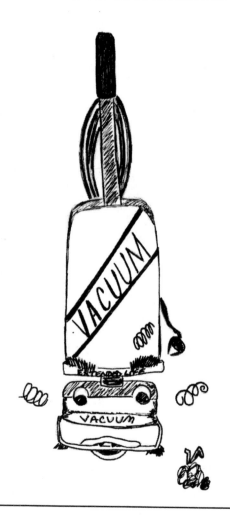

After the three weeks of hell I went through waiting for test results etc., my oncologist finally called. We went over my results, my staging and the form of treatment I should undertake. I was relieved, not by the news of cancer but that I had a starting point. I had somewhere to begin fighting. Believe it or not I became overwhelmed with energy. So much so I vigorously started cleaning the house. Oh and believe me it needed it. Remember for three weeks I was in my own world. Nothing got done and I didn't care. Let's get back to the cleaning issue. I vacuumed the house so much that my muscles ached for three days. My bathroom was so clean the kids could have had breakfast on the tile floor. And believe me the bathroom in my house can get dirty. Especially, my husband and son, they have issues with aiming. You know. They both need target practice. The place was gleaming. My mother thought I hired a cleaning lady. So as a result I had advanced breast cancer but my house was clean. My point, cleaning can be very therapeutic. Just to note, my house has never been that clean again and hopefully never will be.

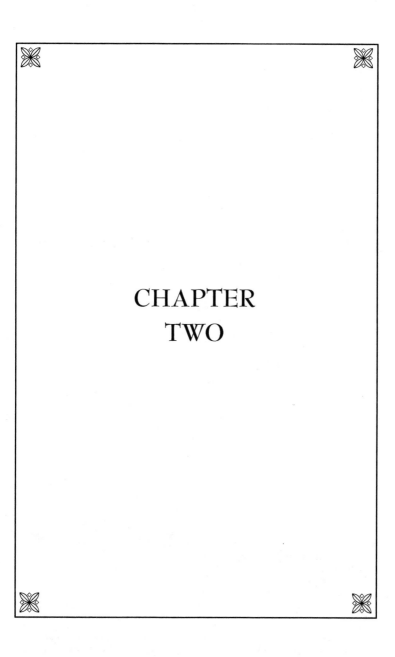

CHAPTER
TWO

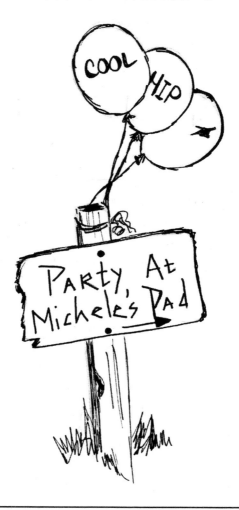

I told my parents the terrible news. My mother was absolutely devastated, which was to be expected. She's a mother and would do anything to help her children. My dad was even worse. He just does not handle crisis well at all. They felt helpless. But I held it together for them. How odd, go figure, I'm the one with cancer. They were so badly distraught that my family members preferred to come to my house than to visit them. My brother told me he didn't want to visit them that I was more fun to be around. My dad was like a raving lunatic yelling profanities as he walked around the house. We're talking about a man who didn't allow us to say "fart" until we were in our twenties. I still don't use that word around him. I'm afraid he might punish me. My mother ran around the house slamming doors and cleaning closets. My brother didn't even want to repeat what she was saying because he couldn't believe his mother would know such words. We thought maybe she was secretly hanging out in biker bars. I thought. Hey I'm not so bad. I'm holding it together better than they are. How great was that? I was somebody just diagnosed with cancer and still was cool and hip to hang out with. I was doing something right. So I figured I'd have a party. And I did because let's not forget I was cool. My point, celebrate life because you're not dead yet!

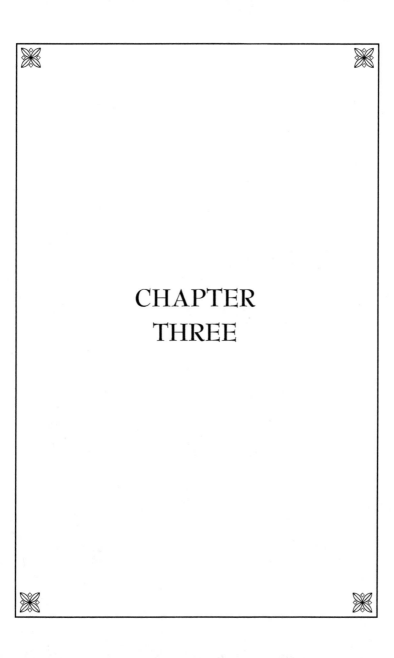

CHAPTER
THREE

CHEMO AND DR. LOVE

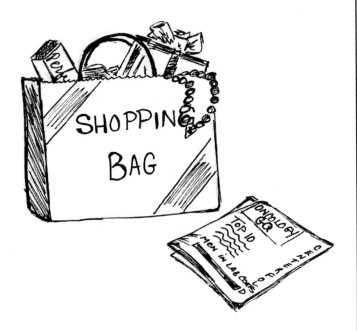

So here I am the "hip cancer patient" starting chemo. The "hip" didn't last too long. It felt like the worst and longest hangover. Words cannot truly describe how horrible it was. But I'll try. It is like your body begins to die and then your slowly brought back to life again. I would actually get anxiety knowing that my treatment was coming up. And just when you thought you had made it through, it was time to do it all over again. I knew that it would only last a few days every time I had a treatment so I thought I need something to look forward to. What not better to do, than shop. I highly recommend it. Your husbands or boyfriends might not but hell you're the one going through chemo. So spend a little money. Just a little advice, don't spend yours, spend theirs. So every two weeks I would hit Bloomingdales. If there was a sale I was there. It was great! Of course my husband had to get a second job but that's O.K. My point, spending money feels wonderful!

Not that I would want anyone to have to find an oncologist but if the need arises, find one that is as wonderful as mine. My doctor is great. And what helps more that he's really intelligent. Oh, all right I'll admit it. He's handsome. Oh, hell let's go for it. He's a little hottie. I love my husband to death but I know a good-looking man when I see one. I won't mention his name but he knows who he is. No disrespect intended but beauty is an art in my book. Obviously you should choose an oncologist who you feel comfortable with, who is experienced, and who would give you the best treatment options. But heck, why not add on looks? Remember it's O.K. to look. Need I finish the rest? So if your going through chemo put on the makeup, brush in the eyebrows. Glue on the eyelashes and don't forget the lipstick. Hell, pretend it's a date. Do what you have to do. Pull yourself together and you might forget what you went to the doctor's office for in the first place. Just don't call him "Dr. Love." I don't think that would go over to well. My point, in some case's looks do matter. Who are we kidding?

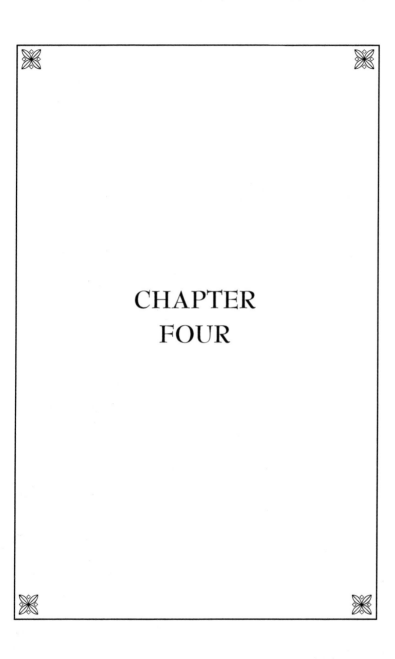

CHAPTER
FOUR

HAIR LOSS

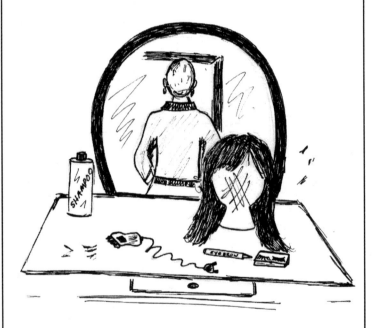

Did I mention after the makeup and glueing on the eyelashes? You might need to put on the hair? In other words purchase a wig. Yes your hair will come out in clumps. I started shedding worse than the dog and cat. I said to my husband, "Honey why is the dog shedding in the summer?" He said, "Honey, it's not the dog it's you." So I gave in and I allowed my husband to shave it all off. My kids watched in laughter. They thought it was the greatest thing to see mommy's hair fall out. They actually would rub my head quite often. So the hair fell to the floor and I calmly walked into the bathroom. I cried my eyes out. Boy did I have an ugly head. That's all I kept thinking. I could no longer be one of those obnoxious women. You know, the ones with the long manes who liked to whip their hair from side to side and take innocent victims eyes out. Anyway, as I cried hysterically, I thought why can't I look like Demi Moore in GI Jane. Dammit she was bald and beautiful in that movie. I know the movie was a flop but she had a body to back it up. And she had a great looking head. Life wasn't fair. My poor husband had issues with me losing my hair. The poor guy was suffering from dandruff so bad. Yes, dandruff. I was to blame. You see, being that I didn't have hair, there was no need to wash my hair. Therefore, there was no reason to buy shampoo. He went months like this without saying a word. I said,

"Why couldn't you use the kids shampoo?" His reply was that, "It was kids' shampoo." It doesn't make any sense to me that you would choose to use dish detergent over children's shampoo. Whatever! Did I feel sorry for him? Hell no! At least he had hair to wash. Well, his dandruff subsided and yes he now buys his own shampoo. I'm so proud of him. My point, if somebody tells you "Oh it will grow back!" Tell them, "Kiss my you know what!"

Buy a wig or wear a hat. That's what it had come to. So with the pressure from friends I bought this beautiful natural hair wig. It looked awesome. You couldn't even tell it wasn't my hair. But no one told me it would cost me a small fortune to purchase. I could have paid off a credit card with the price of this wig. Anyway it looked good. So good it fooled people. They had no idea. So one afternoon I got myself all dolled up. You know the makeup, hair, the works. I ran a few errands and went to the doctors office for my treatment. The building was under construction and there was a bunch of carpenters on lunch break. As I walked up to the building, they started whistling at me, "Hey sweetheart!" So I said to myself, "I can turn heads. I still have it." But then, I got angry. I thought how dare they talk to me that way. I was insulted. I don't know what came over me but in that instant that very moment something happened. I gently lifted my wig and exposed my ugly bald head. Talk about utter shock. It was priceless. They didn't know what to say. It sure wasn't, "Hey baby!" So off to treatment I went. My point, I still have it!

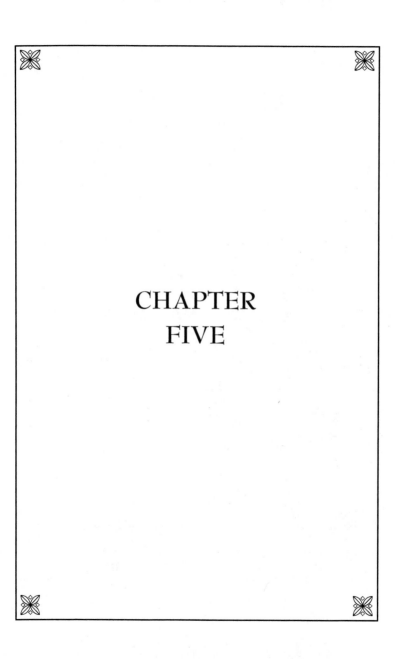

CHAPTER
FIVE

THE BOOB THING

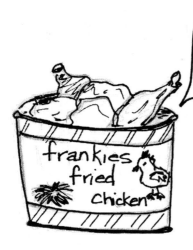

Let's get back to Demi Moore and her awesome body. Plastic surgery. No plastic surgery. I was jealous. You see, I knew my body would be changing very soon. I had chosen to have a double mastectomy. And to be very honest the surgery wasn't that bad. It just gave me another reason to go shopping. God help my husband. So off to the hospital I went. The drugs were great. It would be wonderful if you could have an emergency supply at home just for those moments when needed. You know kids acting up, husband making you angry, inlaws driving you crazy? Just pop a couple of those and you're home free. Anyway, the funny thing was while in the hospital for my surgery, I had this incredible urge for fried chicken breast. It was so bad that my husband went searching for some on a Sunday afternoon. Of course my mom, sister and I had to convince him to go. So we started chanting, "I want breasts, I want breasts!" The nurses thought we were crazy. He eventually went but to our disappointment everything was closed. We settled for cheese steaks. I will never look at chicken breast in the same way again. Who would have thought that? I would envy a chicken and her breasts. Speaking of breasts or the lack of them, I remember something that helped me through the shock of losing them. You see, once you tell somebody you have breast cancer the first thing they do is look at your breasts. Are they there, are they not there? It becomes annoying. You almost feel like flashing them but for some of us there is nothing to flash. So I had an idea. I wanted a Hooters T-shirt. My brother brought one back for me from a business trip from Austin, Texas. Nobody thought I would wear it. Oh, how they were wrong! Talk about confusion. A boobless woman wearing a Hooters T-shirt? I'm surprised the company didn't sue me for false advertisement. I do have to admit I still wear the shirt around the house. My husband even looks confused. But like he always says, "I'm not a boob man, I'm a butt man." Gotta love him, but he's a terrible liar. My point, keep a firm ass!

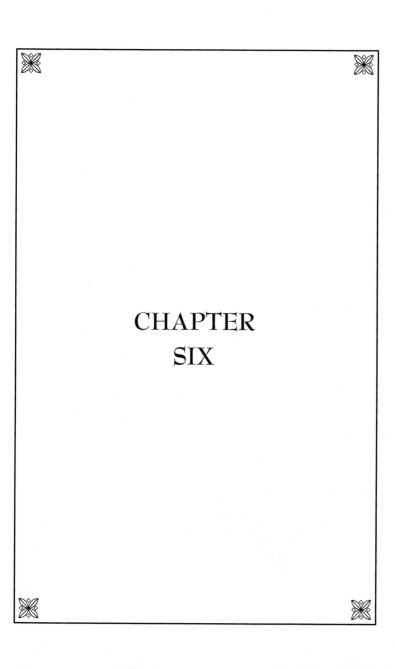

CHAPTER
SIX

VANITY, RECONSTRUCTION
AND TATTOOS

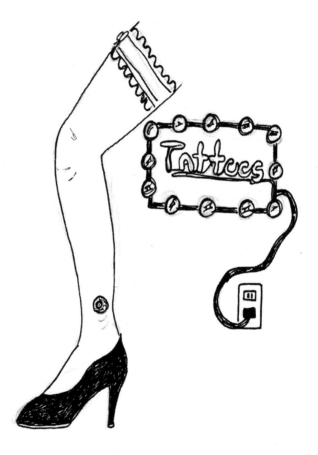

I never thought of getting a tattoo until the issue of nipples came up with my plastic surgeon. Who would have thought, they could actually tattoo nipples to your new reconstructed breasts. Wow, I thought, "Maybe he took classes in the finer art of tattooing." Who knows? Not only could I have my nipples done but I could maybe have a cartoon character tattooed on my ankle. You know nothing too big of course. So I figured why not ask. I was misinformed. Well not completely. I could have a tattoo on my ankle, back, anywhere within reason. The only catch was that they would be nipples. Let's see? I'd wake up from surgery with nipples tattooed all over my body. I don't think so. I found out he doesn't do Botox parties either. I really think he should reconsider. I could make him a lot of money. I know a lot of ladies with a lot of lines, who have a lot of money! My point, make sure your nipples are tattooed to your new breasts and not your ankles.

Vanity comes into question obviously when deciding to have mastectomies. But before I go any further I like to make myself clear. Everyone should make their own decisions! I don't want to ruffle any feathers. Due to a complication I had to postpone my reconstruction and have my implants removed. And I later decided not to have reconstruction at all. I guess you can say. I can fake it pretty well. Actually I didn't want any more surgeries, at least for a while. I'm O.K. with whom I am now and maybe down the road I'll change my mind. But for now I'm faking it. Anyway, I hope that women make their decisions based on how they fell about their body and not what everybody else will think. Most importantly husbands. Your choice should be yours. It's your body. And if your partner truly loves you, it shouldn't matter. Now maybe I've made some people angry by saying this. My point, is that it should be your decision and not pressure from others. This includes doctors because when your first diagnosed there is a lot going on. Make wise choices that are yours. Now enough of the seriousness, on a more humorous note. Being that I chose not to have reconstruction, I now have prosthetic boobs. I can be whatever size I want any day of the week. But the down side is, I have to make sure they're not crooked. There's nothing worse than lop sided boobs. Especially, when your mom has to tell you, "Honey, I think you need to adjust yourself." So there you are fixing you boobs in the middle of the supermarket. My point, if you need an adjustment, go to the garage.

*

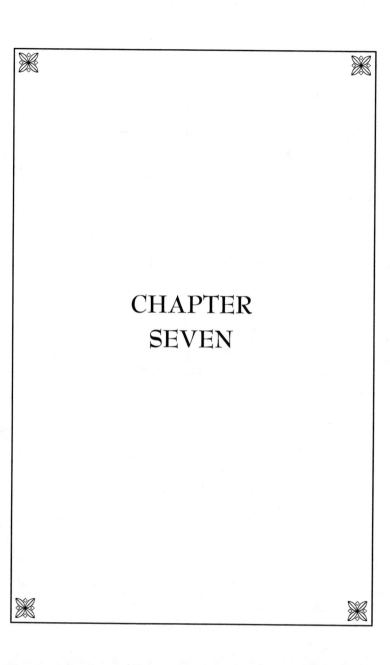

CHAPTER
SEVEN

NUTRITION

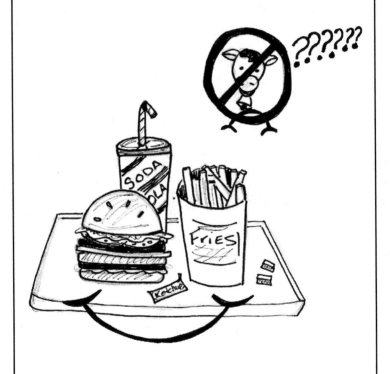

Obviously, nutrition has a big factor with getting well and feeling healthy. The more research I did, the more confused I got. One thing I was sure of was to stay clear of soy and eat a lot of broccoli. So I would cut out Chinese Food and become the poster child on how important it was to eat your "greens." I wasn't really sure about meat. Meat or no meat. That was the question. I decided to cut it out completely. I'm not telling anyone that this is what you have to do. Again,

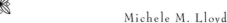

everyone should make their own decisions on what's best for them. So here I am the converted vegetarian. I had no idea what to eat. I was definitely getting sick of spaghetti. Let's face it. I was absolutely starving. I hated buying the kids Mc Donald's. Yes, I know they have salads now. But come on, do you know what torture it is to go to Mc Donald's and eat salad? Get real! For God"s sake it's Mc Donald's. Anyway, I was proud of myself. I only ate the french fries. Here is what put me over the edge. As time went by, I met more women that were vegetarians and also had been diagnosed with breast cancer. So, I did a survey and most of them were vegetarians before they were diagnosed with cancer. Ah hah! A small crack in my vegetarian wall. My wheels started to turn. Is it possible that I can go back to eating delicious hamburgers, wonderful steaks, heck even my Mom's horrible meatloaf? I still wasn't quite sure until I met this great girl at a support group meeting. She was beautiful and was a pilates instructor. Most important, she was a breast cancer survivor that had been a vegetarian almost all of her life. That's all I needed to hear. Halelugah! My point, there is nothing like a Big Mac and don't forget the fries!

CHAPTER
EIGHT

SUPPORT GROUPS

As soon as I was diagnosed with cancer, I was told by many people to find a support group. I thought, "Why do I need to talk to a bunch of women about the possibility of dying for? I didn't need to add to my depression! But I succumbed to the pressure and went anyway. I could have never have been so wrong. The group of women that I met are absolutely wonderful. They welcomed me with open arms. They took me under their wings. They taught me things I could have never had dreamed of. You see. We didn't just talk about cancer. We discussed everything. And I mean everything. They informed me and not discretely I must say that my body would be changing from the many medications I was taking or would be taking. Anyway, let's just say they had a never-ending knowledge of the use of K-Y jelly and many other lubricants. I couldn't believe it! They new what worked, what didn't work, and even what warmed up. I thought what a bunch of sex crazed maniacs. Heck, I admit it, I was jealous. I told my husband. He thought I should definitely keep going back. Yeah, I wonder what he was thinking. You see, when it comes down to it we're like a bunch of old hens in a chicken house. And I'm proud to be a chick. My point, find a support group. Oh, and by the way, lubricants are good.

Being a part of a support group, I learned about many fund-raisers dinners and walks for breast cancer. I knew that there would be a three-mile walk organized by the support group that I was a part of. It was three weeks after my surgery. I decided I would do it with my family and kids. How hard could it be? It was only three miles. So we all got up bright and early one Sunday morning. I was excited that I was doing something for a cause. The walk started out well. My family was at my side. Our banner was flying. I noticed that my husband and the rest of my family were walking too fast. It wasn't a marathon. It was a walk. So I made my husband stay with me and the rest moved on. I was insulted. This was my walk. How dare they leave me. Anyway, my son was in his carriage and my daughter was at my side. I thought, "I didn't think it was going to get so hot out its October." I started shedding my clothing. My daughter kept telling me to hurry up. This was harder than I thought. Sweat was poring off of me. My husband asked me if I was O.K. I yelled at him, "I'm fine!" Anyway, I was a trooper I finished the walk and my family was waiting for me at the finish line. Little did they know that after about the second mile I threw my three-year-old son out of the carriage. Yes, I'm ashamed to say it. I got in the carriage and made my husband push me. I got out before the finish line with a smile on my face as if I had just won the Boston marathon. It was a proud moment. I wasn't gonna tell. I guess it's out now. Doesn't matter. I already collected the sponsor donations! My point, get the money first!

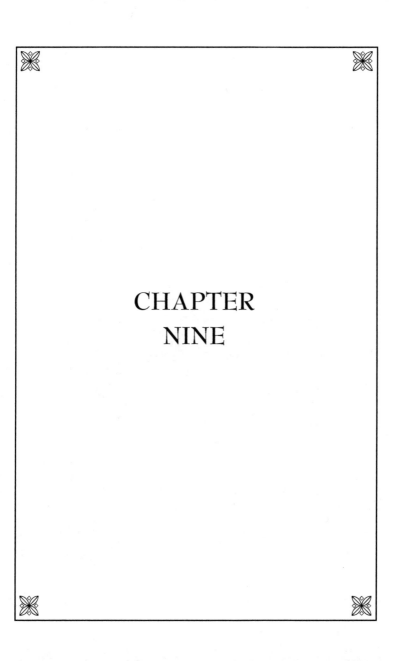

CHAPTER
NINE

Keeping Up With The Jones'

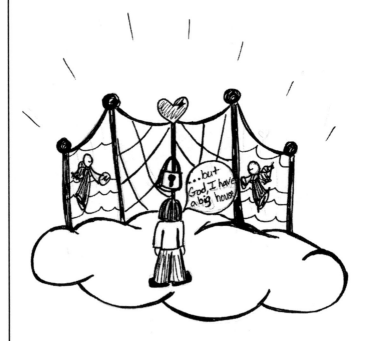

I never realized that I was heading in the wrong direction in my life until I got cancer. What I mean is that I thought I was living the normal life. You know great husband, beautiful kids, pretty house, nice cars and vacation once a year. All the amenities. I was always striving for more. Never really appreciating what I already had. Then I was diagnosed with cancer. And I realized what a selfish ass I was. I don't mean that I was a bad person but I obviously was becoming more focused on what

I didn't have than what I did have. Now I'm not saying that everybody should get cancer to realize how truly blessed they are. But when I truly think about it, for me, it would have taken that no matter what. Throughout our lives we hear about a family member, friends etc., being sick or someone who has passed. And we say "Oh how terrible or awful." And we go about our business. It doesn't really hit home or register. Not that we don't care but it's not as deep rooted. Something happened to me when I was told I had breast cancer. I changed as a person. I don't feel quite the same as your average Joe. I feel blessed by this and at times lonely too. It's a double-edged sword. I see the world differently. I know what it feels like to truly worry about dying and leaving my family. But with this comes a gift. And that is the gift of showing people or teaching people the value of life. I wish I could take anyone by the hand and let them feel the fear of dying so that they would appreciate the beautiful gifts they already have. Maybe I can inspire people to do more with their lives. I don't think I'm some super hero now but I know in my heart that there is some other meaning and purpose as to why this happened to me. My point, who cares how big your house is. What matters is how big your heart is. Square footage doesn't get you into heaven.

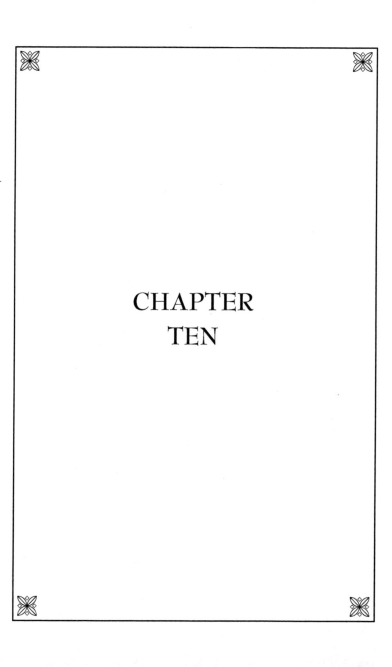

CHAPTER
TEN

FEELING SORRY FOR YOURSELF

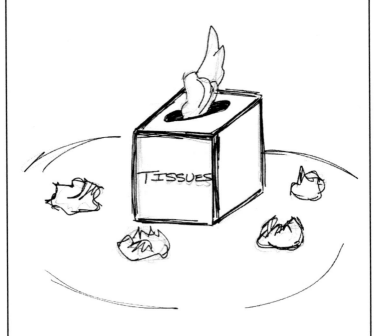

We all have felt sorry for ourselves in one way or another. But I never go there now. And I can honestly say that. It will do absolutely nothing for you but keep you from moving on. This is what keeps me moving on and maybe this I hope will help you. Along my journey I have met many wonderful people. But the one young woman that stands out is amazing. So if you are feeling down, and feel like you don't know how you're going to make it through, think of her. I won't mention her name but I'll tell you a little bit about her.

This young mom is a great gal. I met her during my radiation treatments. She was always so jolly and friendly. Every day she would come into the treatment locker room. We would gather and chat. One day before treatment I had a breakdown. I started to cry on the radiation table. My son had been up the night before sick. And on top of that I had bronchitis. I had been in treatments for a few weeks and was already burnt to a crisp. I just lost it. Of course everyone was wonderful. They were trying to make me feel better. And then I saw my friend in the locker room. She asked me if I was all right. She began to tell me that it's hard when you're really tired from taking care of the kids etc. But then she went on and I really felt like a fool. She told me that her son was eight and was born with severe disabilities. He needed twenty-four hour care. She had to get up every four hours to turn him. Sometimes he would become congested and pneumonia would set in. During the time of her surgery for her breast cancer, he developed pneumonia and was hospitalized. So not only did she have the stress of surgery and recovering, her poor son was in the hospital. During her chemotherapy treatments and recovering from them, she couldn't rest. She needed to take of her son. She never complains. She is always positive. She is my inspiration. I truly look up to her. She is the most kindest and selfless person I have ever met. I only wish I could be half the mother she is. So really try to remember that. It does help. Take your experience and let it inspire you to do great things. I don't mean that you have to become someone famous or even save the world. If you can inspire or change someone's life for the better than cancer was worth having. Because, when it is your time to leave the earth, it's not how much you have, it's how much you loved. And whose life you made better. My point, it's all about giving.

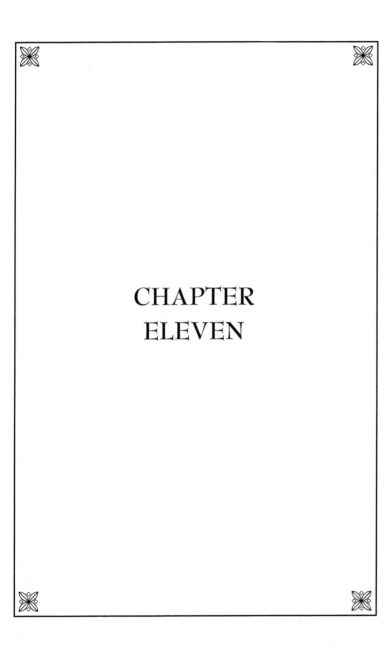

CHAPTER
ELEVEN

PUSHING UP THE DAISIES

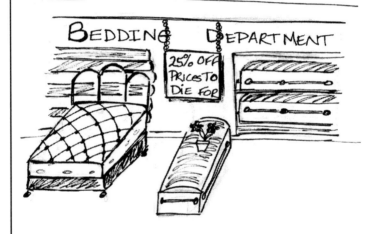

As I mentioned early, when your first diagnosed with cancer you worry about dying. That thought never seems to go away. You learn to live with it every day. So you take every day for all it's worth. Believe it or not I found humor in this as well. One Sunday afternoon as I was thinking about "pushing up the daisies," I saw an article in the paper. It was for an advertisement for a local wholesale club. They were selling caskets in their bedding department. The advertisement said, "prices to die for." Well I thought how tacky, funny and morbid at the same time. I just had to tell my husband and fill him in on the do's and don'ts of buying a casket. Well, actually I screamed at him, "If you ever buy me a casket from the wholesale club, let alone the bedding department, I will come back from the dead and kick your !!**##!!" Just imagine your husband going to the local wholesale club for his wife's casket. What a cheap S.O.B.! I was thinking more in the lines of Gucci, Coach, even Louis Vuitton. Hell, it's my life insurance. Shouldn't it be spent on me? Of course I have no plans on going anywhere. It would be nice at least to have a Louis Vuitton handbag. My point, have a life insurance policy that you can cash in early!

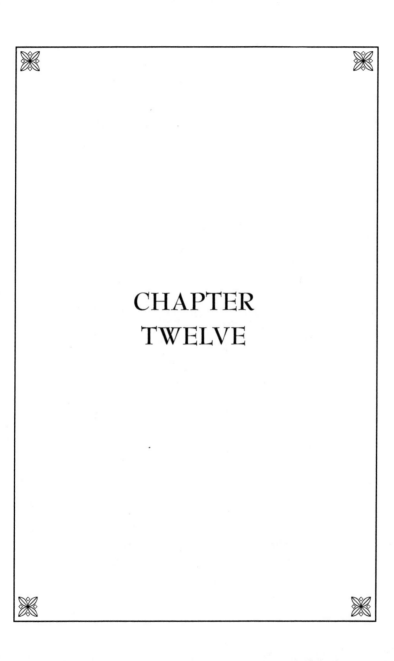

CHAPTER
TWELVE

RADIATION

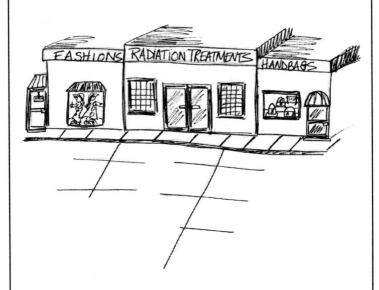

Iknew that after chemotherapy and surgery I would need several weeks of radiation. What a bummer when I found out it was five days a week. At least I had the weekends off. So I made an appointment to meet the radiation oncologist. I called and got directions. As I made my way to the office, I was elated. I couldn't believe it. I was the luckiest radiation patient ever. All right, somewhat lucky. Across the street from the medical building was the local super center How convenient, every day I'd get zapped then shop. And this place had prices to die for! Unfortunately, it wasn't Macy's or Bloomingdale's but at least they had a lay away program. You know beggars can't be choosers. I'd save a little money and make my husband happy about my shopping venture. My point, when deciding where to go for radiation treatments, think location, location, location!

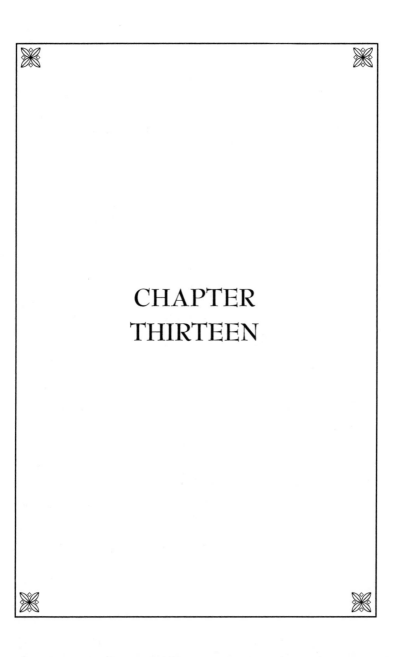

CHAPTER
THIRTEEN

LEARNING HOW TO HAVE FUN AGAIN

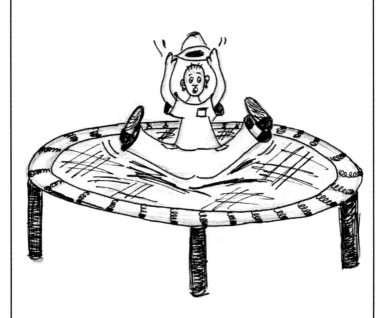

Sometimes with all the doctor's appointments, treatments, surgeries etc., you forget to have fun. Sometimes you're even afraid to have fun. You are so used to being scared or worried. So my advice to all of you who want to find the child inside, buy a trampoline. Yes, I said, "trampoline." And no I'm not crazy. Well maybe just a little. My husband and I bought one for our kids. We thought it would be fun for them. Besides it was exercise. Well they loved it. My daughter convinced me one afternoon to try it out. Of course I looked around to see if the neighbors were watching. It was clear. So I gave it a try. I bounced around for a little while and felt as free as a bird. It was awesome. Of course this was during the time I was still getting chemo treatments so I had to make sure my hat didn't fall off. I didn't want to scare the neighbors. My Mom came over and saw us jumping around. She said, "What the hell are you doing? You're going to break your neck!" I said, "Oh come on Mom, try it out. It will make you feel young again!" So she looked around and whispered, "Are the neighbors watching?" It was all clear. So she climbed up. It was an awesome sight. Three generations hopping around like Jack Rabbits on a trampoline. Until, the neighbors pulled in next door. Well, down we all went. "Did they see?" my Mom yelled. "No but I did!"my husband yelled laughing. So he climbed up as well. But he's a show off and had to out do everybody else. He started doing somersaults. He was pretty good too. My daughter thought her Dad was great. My son was afraid his Dad would trample him. I do have to mention. I have a little secret. He did miss work for two days after that. You see. He pulled a muscle with his acrobatic display. But I'm not supposed to tell. And he says he's not getting old. My point, stretch first!

CHAPTER
FOURTEEN

Fear

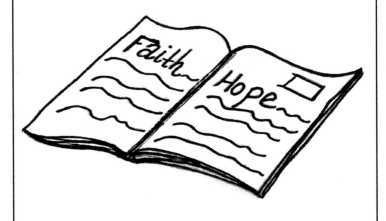

There are a lot of people that ask me how I stay positive. I thought about it. Not only is it my faith, but it's the choice to not curl up and die. Out of everything I have written or have done, this is the most important advice I could give anyone. Fear is evil and not of God. It can take over your life or even take it away. Fear is unhealthy. You need to make a choice whether to fight it or not. This is what works for me and what you should try to do. Get ready for battle. You are a soldier.

Put full body armor on. Stand in front of the mirror. Look fear right in the eyes. Tell fear that you are going to kick its ass! You have control over your mind and soul. Do you want to succumb to fear? No! So move on and pick yourself up. Today is a new day. I'm a part of this day. Nobody with or without cancer is promised tomorrow. I say this often. Hell, we could walk outside, get hit by a bus and not even have to worry about cancer. My point, enjoy life, you're still here!

I know that cancer is absolutely devastating. Not only to the person diagnosed but to their family and friends as well. It is a life changing experience. But rather than to take it as doom and gloom, I choose to take it as something good. I take it as a sign that I need to pay attention to all the beautiful things in my life. I consider myself blessed now. I can look at life more differently than most people. I don't take one minute for granted.

The world is beautiful and most of us miss out on it. You don't need to be a world traveler to see the beauty in it. Just look around where you are right now and there is beauty in everything. My faith guides me and I intend on being a survivor. I can't answer why people die. I'm not God. But I look at it this way. It's like your free falling and you have to know in your heart that know matter what any doctor says to you, God will catch you. It is blind faith. Hebrews 11:1, Now faith is being sure of what we hope for and certain of what we do not see.

My entire point, for all you ladies diagnosed with breast cancer. It's not about the boobs! They're over rated. It's about life!

Things That I Am Grateful For

God
My Beautiful Children
My Selfless Husband
My Family Who Loves Me
Rainbows
Windy Days
Autumn Leaves
Warm Covers On Chilly Mornings
Finding Two Socks That Match From the Laundry Basket.
My Family Pets, Who Tend To Forget that They Are Not Human.
Bacon Cheeseburgers
McDonalds French Fries
Sleeping Late On Saturday Mornings
Watching My Kids Sleep
Finding Jeans That I Can Button
Every Day That I Am Alive

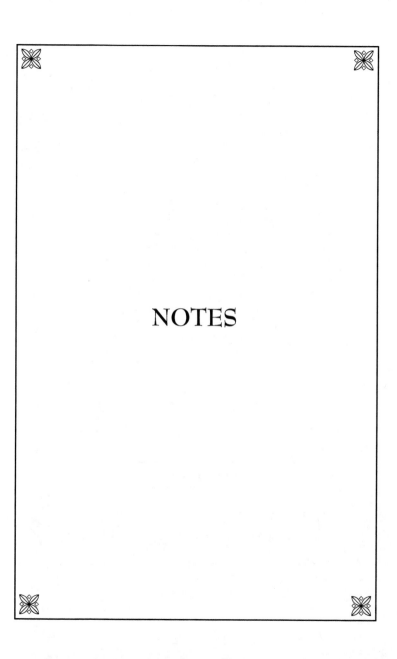

NOTES

Michele M. Lloyd

_____

_____

_____

_____

_____

_____

_____

_____

_____

_____

_____

_____

_____

_____

_____

_____

_____

_____

_____

_____

_____

_____

_____

_____

_____

_____

_____

_____

_____

_____

_____

_____

_____

_____

_____

_____

_____

_____

_____

_____

_____

_____

_____

_____

_____

_____

_____

_____

_____

_____

_____

_____

_____

_____

_____

_____

_____

_____

_____

_____

_____

_____

It's Not About the Boobs

_____

_____

_____

_____

_____

_____

_____

_____

_____

_____

_____

_____

_____

_____

_____

_____

_____

_____

_____

_____

_____

_____

_____

_____

_____

_____

_____

_____

_____

_____

_____

_____

_____

_____

_____

_____

_____

_____

_____

_____

_____

_____

_____

_____

_____

_____

_____

_____

_____

_____

_____

_____

_____

_____

_____

_____

_____

_____

_____

_____

_____

_____

_____

_____

_____

_____

_____

_____

_____

_____

_____

_____

_____

_____

_____

_____

_____

_____

_____

_____

_____

_____

_____

_____

_____

_____

_____

_____

_____

_____

_____

_____

_____

_____

_____

_____

_____

_____

_____

_____

_____

_____

_____

_____

_____

_____

_____

_____

_____

_____

_____

_____

_____

_____

_____

_____

_____

_____

_____

_____

_____

_____

_____

_____

_____

_____

_____

_____

_____

_____

_____

_____

_____

_____

_____

_____

_____

_____

_____

_____

_____

_____

ISBN 141206983-1

9 781412 069830